Pressure Cooker Tasty Recipes for Family

The best collection of Pressure Cooker recipes

Linda C. Welch

Sommario

Introduction..**9**

Dinner...**11**

Seafood Paella & Chorizo **11**

Chili Salmon with Lime **14**

Smoked Shrimp, Sausage and Peppers **16**

Cedar Salmon **19**

Crispy Cod...**21**

Tilapia Fillets with Arugula **23**

The Best Jambalaya Ever **25**

Creamy Cheesy Shrimp Salad **27**

Mom's Halibut Stew 29

Herbed Cod Steaks..32

Warm Tuna Salad..34

Trout Casserole with Pepper-Jack Cheese 36

Buttery and Lemony Tuna Fillets 38

Easy Scallops with Parsley and Wine 40

Aromatic Mahi-Mahi Filets with Peppers......................42

Simple Garlicky Halibut Steak......................................45

Faster-than-Fast-Food Salmon Burgers 47

Basil Wine Scallops..49

Foil-Packet Haddock with Veggies 51

Favorite Monkfish Stew 53

Creole Lobster with Lime Cream Sauce 55

Beer-Poached Alaskan Cod 58

Haddock and Cheese Stuffed Peppers 60

Authentic Garam Masala Fish 62

Red Curry Perch Fillets 64

Bluefish in Tarragon-Vermouth Sauce 66

King Crab with Baby Bellas 68

Simply Creole Sea Scallops 71

Salmon Steaks with Garlic Yogurt 73

Hangover Seafood Bowl 75

Mussels with Tomatoes and White Wine......................77

Scampi Shrimp...79

Creamy Shrimp 80

Paella Pronto with Shrimp and Scallop 83

Fish Tacos...85

Clam Soup...87

Tostadas with Fish and Pineapple...........................89

Scallops and Tomato-Herb Sauce.............................91

Fish Stew 93

Mussels Frites..96

Fish and Greens with Miso Butter 98

Cod with Panko-Crusted 100

Low Country Shrimp 102

Soy-Ginger Dressing Salmon and Broccoli 104

Tomato Cod Fillets with Zucchini 106

Zucchini and Vegetable Tian 109

Tabbouleh Vegetable Quinoa 111

Vegan Chili with 3 Beans 112

Conclusion .... Errore. Il segnalibro non è definito.

Introduction

Considering the principle of diet in current times are based upon fasting, instead our keto instant pot is based upon the extreme decrease of carbs.

This kind of diet is based on the intake of specific foods that allow you to slim down faster permitting you to slim down approximately 3 kg each week.

You will certainly see how simple it will be to make these tasty meals with the tools available as well as you will certainly see that you will certainly be satisfied.

If you are reluctant concerning this fantastic diet plan you simply have to try it as well as analyze your results to a short time, trust me you will be pleased.

Bear in mind that the most effective method to reduce weight is to analyze your situation with the help of a specialist.

Dinner

Seafood Paella & Chorizo

Ingredients for 6 servings:

4 tablespoons olive oil 1 pound cured Spanish chorizo cut into 1 inch thick slices 1 yellow onion diced 3 cloves garlic minced salt pepper freshly ground 2 teaspoons smoked paprika 1 teaspoon sweet paprika ½ teaspoon granulated garlic ½ teaspoon saffron threads ½ cup dry white wine 14 ounces crushed tomatoes with juice 2 cups Basmati rice 4 ¼ cups chicken broth 1 pound littleneck clams or other small clams ¾ pounds large shrimp peeled and deveined with tails intact 1 ½ cups frozen peas flat-leaf parsley chopped fresh, for serving lemon wedges for serving

Directions and total time – 15-30 m

• Select Sauté on the Instant Pot and warm 2 tablespoons of the oil. Add the chorizo and cook, stirring occasionally, until lightly browned and warmed through, about 4 minutes. Transfer the chorizo to a plate. • Warm the remaining 2 tablespoons oil in the pot. Add the onion and minced garlic and cook, stirring occasionally, until the onion is tender and translucent, about 3 minutes. • Season with salt and pepper, then add the smoked paprika, sweet paprika, granulated garlic, and saffron. • Cook, stirring often, until the onion is well coated with the spices, about 3 minutes. Pour in the wine and, using a wooden spoon, scrape up any browned bits from the pot bottom. • Add the tomatoes, rice, 4 cups of the broth, and the clams, discarding any clams that fail to close to the touch. • Lock the lid in place and turn the valve to Sealing. Press the Keep Warm/Cancel button to reset the program, then press the Manual/Pressure Cook button and set the cook time for 8 minutes at high pressure. • Turn the valve to Venting to manually release the steam. When the steam stops, carefully remove the lid, press the Keep Warm/ Cancel button to reset the program, then select Sauté. • Add the remaining ½ cup broth, the shrimp, and the peas and cook, stirring occasionally, until the shrimp are opaque throughout, about 5 minutes. ● Divide the paella among individual bowls, discarding any clams that failed to open. Top with parsley and a squeeze of lemon juice and serve.

Chili Salmon with Lime

Ingredients for 2 servings:

Sauce Mixture: 1 jalapeno seeds removed, diced 2 cloves garlic minced 1 tbsp fresh parsley chopped 1 tbsp lime juice 1 tbsp olive oil 1 tbsp honey 1 tbsp Water ½ tsp paprika ½ tsp cumin ½ tsp lime zest For Fish: 2 salmon fillets 5 ounces each or trout or snapper 1 cup Water ½ tsp kosher salt ⅛ tsp pepper

Directions and total time – 15-30 m • Combine Sauce Mixture ingredients in a large liquid measuring cup or other bowl with a spout. Set aside. • Pour 1 cup of water in the Instant Pot and insert the trivet. • Season the salmon filets with salt and pepper and place them on the trivet. • Secure the lid, making sure the vent is closed. • Using the display panel select the STEAM function. Use the +/- buttons and program the Instant Pot for 5 minutes. • When the time is up, quick-release the remaining pressure. • Serve the salmon with the sauce drizzled over the top.

Smoked Shrimp, Sausage and Peppers

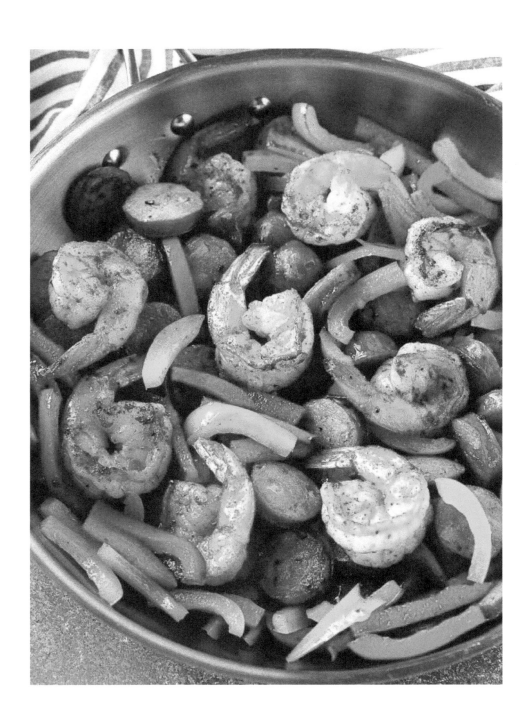

Ingredients for 4 servings:

1 tbsp olive oil 1 small yellow onion peeled and diced ½ green bell pepper seeded and thinly sliced ½ red bell pepper seeded and thinly sliced ½ yellow bell pepper seeded and thinly sliced 14.5 ounces diced tomatoes 1 can including juice 2 lbs large uncooked shrimp peeled and deveined 12 ounces smoked sausage sliced into ½ inch sections 2 tsp Old Bay seasoning ½ tsp salt ½ tsp ground black pepper 1 cup Water

Directions and total time – 15 m

• Combine beer, water, and garlic in the pot. Stir to combine. • Add corn, potatoes and sausage. Sprinkle the cajun seasoning (if using) and 1 tbsp of the Old Bay and over the top. • Secure the lid, making sure the vent is closed. • Using the display panel select the MANUAL or PRESSURE COOK function. Use the +/- buttons and program the Instant Pot for 4 minutes. • When the time is up, quick-release the remaining pressure. • Add shrimp and sprinkle lemon juice and remaining 1 tbsp Old Bay over the top. Replace the lid and make sure the pot is still set to WARM. The residual heat will cook the shrimp. Check for doneness after 5 minutes. • Use a slotted spoon to remove corn, potatoes, sausage and shrimp to a serving platter. • Mix together butter and garlic powder. Pour butter mixture over the platter or serve on the side for dipping. • Garnish with additional Old Bay and/or cajun seasoning. Serve warm.

Cedar Salmon

Ingredients for 2-4 servings:

1 tbsp grainy mustard 1 tbsp honey or maple syrup 1 ½ tsp minced fresh rosemary 1 tbsp lemon juice ½ tsp each kosher salt and pepper 12-16 oz thick-cut salmon Cedar grilling plank sized to fit your Instant Pot (4" x 7" x ¼" works well) Lemon slices

Directions and total time – 15-30 m

• In a small bowl, combine mustard, honey or maple syrup, rosemary, lemon juice, salt and pepper. • Lay the fish, skin side down, on the cedar plank and brush with the mustard mixture. • Pour one cup of water in the Instant Pot and insert the steam rack. Carefully lower the cedar plank on to the steam rack. • Secure the lid, making sure the vent is closed. • Using the display panel select the MANUAL function. Use the +/- keys and program the Instant Pot for 5 minutes. • When the time is up, quick-release the remaining pressure. • Check the fish for desired doneness, and add an additional 1-2 minutes if needed. • Serve hot topped with lemon slices, alongside steamed vegetables or rice (optional).

_____

Crispy Cod

Ingredients for 4 servings:

½ cup flour ½ tsp paprika 1 egg beaten ¼ cup mayonnaise 4 oz salt and vinegar potato chips 1 lb cod fillets or haddock or pollock Tartar sauce and lemon wedges for serving

Directions and total time – 15-30 m

• Place the salt and vinegar potato chips in a ziplock bag and use a rolling pin or mallet to crush to the consistency of panko bread crumbs. • Set up for dredging: Combine flour and paprika in a shallow dish. Combine beaten egg and mayonnaise in a second shallow dish. Add crushed potato chips to a third shallow dish. • Cut fish into 6 pieces. Dredge fish first in the flour mixture, then in the egg mixture, then place the chicken in the potato chip mixture and press the crumbs firmly on both sides. • Divide the coated fish onto the cooking trays, leaving space between each fish piece. • Place the drip pan in the bottom of the cooking chamber.

Using the display panel, select AIRFRY, then adjust the temperature to 370 degrees and the time to 10 minutes, then touch START. • When the display indicates "Add Food" insert one cooking tray in the top-most position and one tray in the bottom-most position. • When the display indicates "Turn Food" switch the cooking trays so that the one that was in the top-most position is now in the bottom-most position, and vice-versa (it is not necessary to flip the fillets). • When the AirFry program is complete, remove the fillets and serve hot with tartar sauce and lemon wedges (optional).

Tilapia Fillets with Arugula

(Ready in about 10 minutes | Servings 4)

Per serving: 145 Calories; 4.9g Fat; 2.4g Carbs; 23.3g Protein; 1.1g Sugars

Ingredients

1 lemon, juiced 1 pound tilapia fillets 2 teaspoons ghee Sea salt and ground black pepper, to taste 1/2 teaspoon cayenne pepper, or more to taste 1/2 teaspoon dried basil 2 cups arugula

Directions

Add fresh lemon juice and 1 cup of water to the bottom of your Instant Pot. Add a metal steamer insert. Brush the fish fillets with melted ghee. Season the fish with salt, black pepper, cayenne pepper; arrange the tilapia fillets in the steamer insert; sprinkle dried basil on top of the fish. Secure the lid. Choose "Manual" mode and Low pressure; cook for 4 minutes. Once cooking is complete, use a quick pressure release; carefully remove the lid. Serve with fresh arugula and enjoy!

_____

The Best Jambalaya Ever

(Ready in about 25 minutes | Servings 6)

Per serving: 351 Calories; 12.1g Fat; 8.9g Carbs; 49g Protein; 3.9g Sugars

Ingredients

2 teaspoons olive oil 1 pound chicken breasts, boneless, skinless and cubed 1 cup smoked sausage, chopped 3/4 pound prawns 1 teaspoon Creole seasoning Sea salt and ground black pepper, to taste 1/2 cup onion, chopped 2 cloves garlic, minced 2 bell peppers, chopped 1 habanero pepper, chopped 1 stalk celery, chopped 2 ripe tomatoes, puréed 2 cups vegetable stock 1 tablespoon freshly squeezed lemon juice 1 tablespoon fresh cilantro, chopped

Directions

Press the "Sauté" button to heat up the Instant Pot. Now, heat the olive oil. Now, cook the chicken and sausage until no longer pink. Then, add prawns and cook for 2 minutes more; season the meat with Creole seasoning, salt, and black pepper and reserve. Add the onion, garlic, peppers, celery, tomatoes, and vegetable stock. Secure the lid. Choose "Manual" mode and High pressure; cook for 9 minutes. Once cooking is complete, use a quick pressure release; carefully remove the lid. Now, add the reserved chicken, sausage, and prawns. Seal the lid and allow it to sit for 6 to 7 minutes. Drizzle fresh lemon over each serving and garnish with fresh cilantro. Bon appétit!

Creamy Cheesy Shrimp Salad

(Ready in about 10 minutes | Servings 4)

Per serving: 326 Calories; 15.3g Fat; 4.1g Carbs; 41.9g Protein; 1.9g Sugars

Ingredients

28 ounces shrimp, peeled and deveined 1/2 cup apple cider vinegar 1/2 cup water 1/3 cup mayonnaise 1/4 cup cream cheese 1 celery with leaves, chopped 1 red onion, chopped 1 large-sized cucumber, sliced 1 tablespoon lime juice 2 tablespoons cilantro, roughly chopped

Directions

Toss the shrimp, apple cider vinegar and water in your Instant Pot. Secure the lid. Choose "Manual" mode and Low pressure; cook for 2 minutes. Once cooking is complete, use a quick pressure release; carefully remove the lid. Allow your shrimp to cool completely. Toss the shrimp with the remaining ingredients. Serve this salad well-chilled and enjoy!

___

Mom's Halibut Stew

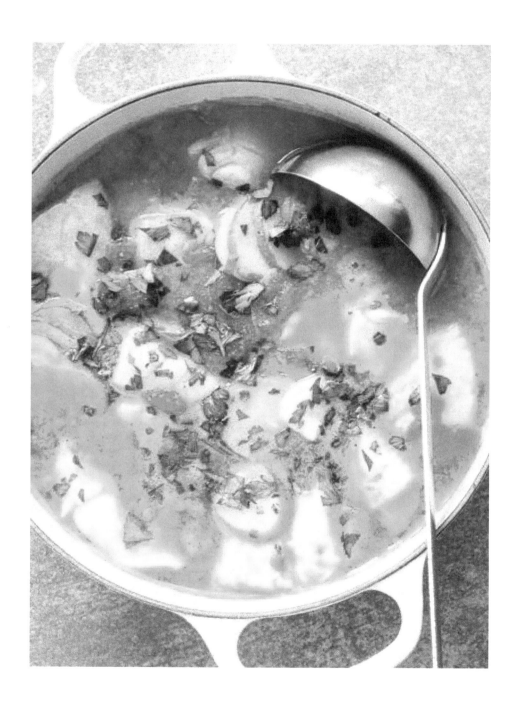

(Ready in about 15 minutes | Servings 4)

Per serving: 432 Calories; 29.9g Fat; 5.4g Carbs; 34.6g Protein; 4.3g Sugars

Ingredients

4 slices bacon, chopped 1/2 cup shallots, chopped 1 teaspoon garlic, smashed 1 celery, chopped 1 parsnip, chopped 2 cups fish stock 1 tablespoon coconut oil, softened 1 pound halibut Sea salt and crushed black peppercorns, to taste 1/4 teaspoon ground allspice 1 cup double cream 1 cup Cottage cheese, at room temperature

Directions

Press the "Sauté" button to heat up the Instant Pot. Now, cook the bacon until it is nice and crispy. Add the shallots, garlic, celery, and parsnip. Continue to sauté for 2 minutes longer or until vegetables are just tender. Stir in the stock, coconut oil, halibut, salt, black peppercorns, and allspice. Secure the lid. Choose "Manual" mode and Low pressure; cook for 7 minutes. Once cooking is complete, use a natural pressure release; carefully remove the lid. After that, stir in double cream and cheese. Press the "Sauté" button again and let it simmer for a couple of minutes or until everything is heated through. Bon appétit!

Herbed Cod Steaks

(Ready in about 10 minutes | Servings 4)

Per serving: 190 Calories; 7.7g Fat; 2.6g Carbs; 26.2g Protein; 1.1g Sugars

Ingredients

4 cod steaks, 1 ½-inch thick 2 tablespoons garlic-infused oil Sea salt, to taste 1/2 teaspoon mixed peppercorns, crushed 1 sprig rosemary 2 sprigs thyme 1 yellow onion, sliced

Directions

Prepare your Instant Pot by adding 1 ½ cups of water and a metal rack to the inner pot. Then, massage the garlic-infused oil into the cod steaks; sprinkle them with salt and crushed peppercorns. Lower the cod steaks onto the rack skin side down; place rosemary, thyme, and onion on the top. Secure the lid. Choose "Manual" mode and High pressure; cook for 4 minutes. Once cooking is complete, use a quick pressure release; carefully remove the lid.

Serve immediately with a fresh salad of choice. Bon appétit!

Warm Tuna Salad

(Ready in about 10 minutes | Servings 4)

Per serving: 163 Calories; 4.7g Fat; 7.4g Carbs; 23.5g Protein; 4.1g Sugars

Ingredients

1 pound tuna steaks 2 Roma tomatoes, sliced 1 red bell pepper, sliced 1 green bell pepper, sliced 1 head lettuce 2 tablespoons Kalamata olives, pitted and halved 1 red onion, chopped 2 tablespoons balsamic vinegar 2 tablespoons extra-virgin olive oil Sea salt, to taste 1/2 teaspoon chili flakes

Directions

Prepare your Instant Pot by adding 1 ½ cups of water and steamer basket to the inner pot. Place the tuna steaks in your steamer basket. Place the tomato slices and bell peppers on top of the fish. Secure the lid. Choose "Manual" mode and High pressure; cook for

4 minutes. Once cooking is complete, use a quick pressure release; carefully remove the lid. Flake the fish with a fork. Divide lettuce leaves among serving plates to make a bad for your salad. Now, add olives and onions. Drizzle balsamic vinegar and olive oil over the salad. Sprinkle salt and chili flakes over your salad. Top with the prepared fish, tomatoes, and bell peppers. Enjoy!

Trout Casserole with Pepper-Jack Cheese

(Ready in about 15 minutes | Servings 3)

Per serving: 408 Calories; 24.2g Fat; 3.6g Carbs; 42.3g Protein; 1.8g Sugars

Ingredients

1 ½ tablespoons olive oil 3 plum tomatoes, sliced 1 teaspoon dried basil 1/2 teaspoon dried oregano 3 trout fillets 1/2 teaspoon cayenne pepper, or more to taste 1/3 teaspoon black pepper Salt, to taste 1 bay leaf 1 cup Pepper-Jack cheese, shredded

Directions

Prepare your Instant Pot by adding 1 ½ cups of water and a metal rack to the bottom of the inner pot. Now, grease a baking dish with olive oil. Place the slices of tomatoes on the bottom of the baking dish. Sprinkle the basil and oregano over them. Now, add fish fillets; season with cayenne pepper, black pepper, and salt. Add bay leaf. Lower the baking dish onto the rack. Secure the lid. Choose "Manual" mode and High pressure; cook for 10 minutes. Once cooking is complete, use a quick pressure release; carefully remove the lid. Lastly, top with Pepper-Jack cheese, seal the lid and allow the cheese to melt. Serve warm. Bon appétit!

Buttery and Lemony Tuna Fillets

(Ready in about 10 minutes | Servings 4)

Per serving: 175 Calories; 6.9g Fat; 1.9g Carbs; 25.2g Protein; 0.3g Sugars

Ingredients

1 cup water 1/3 cup lemon juice 2 sprigs fresh rosemary 2 sprigs fresh thyme 2 sprigs fresh parsley 1 pound tuna fillets 4 cloves garlic, pressed Sea salt, to taste 1/4 teaspoon black pepper, or more to taste 2 tablespoons butter, melted 1 lemon, sliced

Directions

Prepare your Instant Pot by adding 1 cup of water, lemon juice, rosemary, thyme, and parsley to the bottom. Add a steamer basket too. Now, place tuna fillets in the steamer basket. Place the garlic on the top of fish fillets; sprinkle with salt and black pepper. Drizzle the melted butter over the fish fillets and top with the sliced lemon.

Secure the lid. Choose "Manual" mode and Low pressure; cook for 3 minutes. Once cooking is complete, use a quick pressure release; carefully remove the lid. Serve warm and enjoy!

Easy Scallops with Parsley and Wine

(Ready in about 10 minutes | Servings 3)

Per serving: 165 Calories; 7.6g Fat; 5.7g Carbs; 17.6g Protein; 0.3g Sugars

Ingredients

1 tablespoon sesame oil 3/4 pound scallops 2 garlic cloves, crushed Sea salt, to taste 1/3 teaspoon ground black pepper 1/2 teaspoon paprika 1 cup broth, preferably homemade 1/4 cup dry white wine 2 tablespoons fresh parsley, chopped 1 tablespoon fresh lemon juice

Directions

Press the "Sauté" button to heat up the Instant Pot. Now, heat the oil and sauté the scallops for 1 to 2 minutes. Add the garlic and continue to sauté for 30 seconds longer. Add the salt, black pepper, paprika, broth, and wine. Secure the lid. Choose "Manual" mode and Low pressure; cook for 2 minutes. Once cooking is complete, use a quick pressure release; carefully remove the lid. Toss the scallops with fresh parsley and lemon juice. Bon appétit!

Aromatic Mahi-Mahi Filets with Peppers

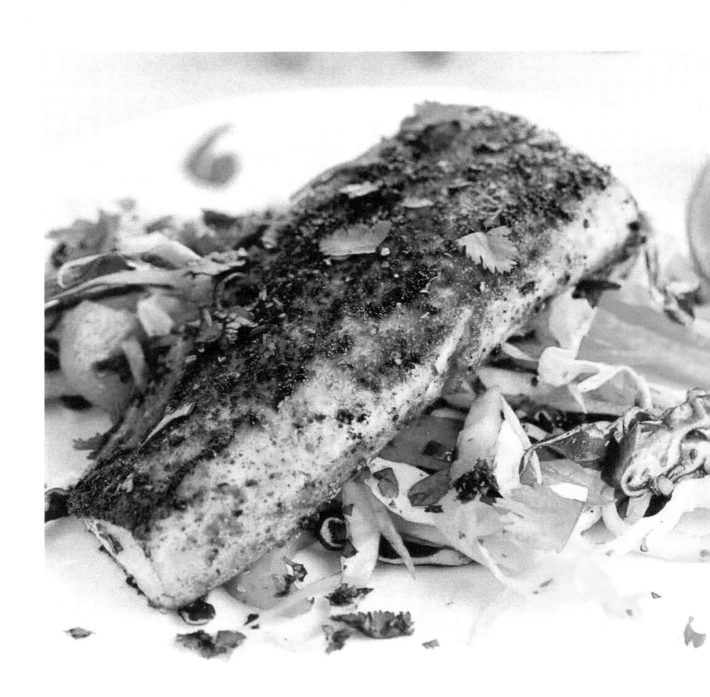

(Ready in about 10 minutes | Servings 3)

Per serving: 205 Calories; 9.8g Fat; 5.4g Carbs; 24.1g Protein; 2.8g Sugars

Ingredients

1 cup water 2 sprigs fresh rosemary 1 sprig fresh thyme 2 sprigs dill, tarragon 1 lemon, sliced 3 mahi-mahi filets 2 tablespoons coconut oil, melted Sea salt and ground black pepper, to taste 1 red bell pepper, sliced 1 green bell pepper, sliced 1 serrano pepper, seeded and sliced

Directions

Add water, herbs, and lemon slices to the Instant Pot; add a steamer basket. Place mahi-mahi filets in the steamer basket. Drizzle mahi-mahi with melted coconut oil; sprinkle with salt and black pepper. Secure the lid. Choose "Manual" mode and Low pressure; cook for 3 minutes. Once cooking is complete, use a natural pressure release; carefully remove the lid. Arrange the peppers on the top of fish fillets. Press the "Sauté" button and let it cook for just 1 minute or so. Serve immediately.

Simple Garlicky Halibut Steak

(Ready in about 10 minutes | Servings 3)

Per serving: 287 Calories; 20.9g Fat; 1.3g Carbs; 21.9g Protein; 0g Sugars

Ingredients

3 halibut steaks 4 garlic cloves, crushed Coarse sea salt, to taste 1/4 teaspoon ground black pepper, to taste

Directions

Prepare your Instant Pot by adding 1 ½ cups of water and steamer basket to the inner pot. Place the halibut steaks in the steamer basket; season them with salt and black pepper. Secure the lid. Choose "Manual" mode and High pressure; cook for 5 minutes. Once cooking is complete, use a quick pressure release; carefully remove the lid. Serve with favorite keto sides. Bon appétit!

Faster-than-Fast-Food Salmon Burgers

(Ready in about 10 minutes | Servings 4)

Per serving: 307 Calories; 18.4g Fat; 2.1g Carbs; 31.9g Protein; 0.9g Sugars

Ingredients

1 pound salmon, boneless and skinless 2 tablespoons scallions, chopped 1 teaspoon garlic, finely minced Sea salt and ground black pepper, to taste 1 teaspoon cayenne pepper 1 teaspoon stone-ground mustard 1 cup Romano cheese, grated 1 tablespoon fresh coriander, chopped 1/2 teaspoon dried dill

Directions

Mix all of the above ingredients in your food processor until everything is well incorporated. Now, shape the mixture into 4 patties and set aside. Prepare your Instant Pot by adding 1 ½ cups of water and steamer basket to the inner pot. Place fish burgers in the steamer basket. Secure the lid. Choose "Manual" mode and Low pressure; cook for 3 minutes. Once cooking is complete, use a quick pressure release; carefully remove the lid. Serve with mayo, lettuce, tomato, and keto buns. Enjoy!

Basil Wine Scallops

(Ready in about 10 minutes | Servings 5)

Per serving: 209 Calories; 10.5g Fat; 8.8g Carbs; 19.2g Protein; 2.6g Sugars

Ingredients

1 tablespoon olive oil 1 brown onion, chopped 2 garlic cloves, minced 1/2 cup port wine 1 ½ pounds scallops, peeled and deveined 1/2 cup fish stock 1 ripe tomato, crushed Sea salt and ground black pepper, to taste 1 teaspoon smoked paprika 2 tablespoons fresh lemon juice 1/2 cup cream cheese, at room temperature 2 tablespoons fresh basil, chopped

Directions

Press the "Sauté" button to heat up your Instant Pot. Now, heat the oil and cook the onion and garlic until fragrant. Add the wine to deglaze the bottom. Add the scallops, fish stock, tomato, salt, black pepper, and paprika. Secure the lid. Choose "Manual" mode and Low pressure; cook for 1 minute. Once cooking is complete, use a quick pressure release; carefully remove the lid. Drizzle fresh lemon juice over the scallops and top them with cream cheese. Cover and let it sit in the residual heat for 3 to 5 minutes. Serve warm garnished with fresh basil leaves, and enjoy!

Foil-Packet Haddock with Veggies

(Ready in about 15 minutes | Servings 4)

Per serving: 180 Calories; 3.9g Fat; 2.4g Carbs; 32g Protein; 1.2g Sugars

Ingredients

1 ½ cups of water 1 lemon, sliced 1 brown onion, sliced into rings 2 bell peppers, sliced 2 sprigs rosemary 4 sprigs parsley 2 sprigs thyme 4 haddock fillets Sea salt, to taste 1/3 teaspoon ground black pepper, or more to taste 2 tablespoons extra-virgin olive oil

Directions

Start by adding water and lemon to your Instant Pot. Now, add a steamer basket. Assemble the packets with large sheets of heavy-duty foil. Mound onions rings, peppers, rosemary, parsley, and thyme in the center of each foil. Place the fish fillet on the top of the vegetables. Season with salt and black pepper, and drizzle with olive oil. Place the packets in the steamer basket. Secure the lid. Choose "Manual" mode and Low pressure; cook for 10 minutes. Once cooking is complete, use a quick pressure release; carefully remove the lid. Serve warm.

Favorite Monkfish Stew

(Ready in about 40 minutes | Servings 6)

Per serving: 163 Calories; 7.6g Fat; 3.4g Carbs; 19.8g Protein; 1.6g Sugars

Ingredients

Juice of 1 lemon 1 tablespoon fresh parsley 1 tablespoon fresh basil 1 teaspoon garlic, minced 1 tablespoon olive oil 1 ½ pounds monkfish 1 tablespoon butter 1 onion, sliced 1 bell pepper, chopped 1/4 teaspoon ground cumin 1/4 teaspoon turmeric powder 1/2 teaspoon cayenne pepper Sea salt and ground black pepper, to taste 2 cups fish stock 1/2 cup water 1/4 cup dry white wine 1 ripe tomato, crushed 2 bay leaves 1/2 teaspoon mixed peppercorns

Directions

In a ceramic dish, whisk the lemon juice, parsley, basil, garlic, and olive oil; add monkfish and let it marinate for 30 minutes. Press the "Sauté" button to heat up your Instant Pot. Now, melt the butter and cook the onion and bell peppers until fragrant. Add the remaining ingredients and gently stir to combine. Secure the lid. Choose "Manual" mode and High pressure; cook for 6 minutes. Once cooking is complete, use a quick pressure release; carefully remove the lid. Afterwards, discard bay leaves and ladle your stew into serving bowls. Serve hot.

Creole Lobster with Lime Cream Sauce

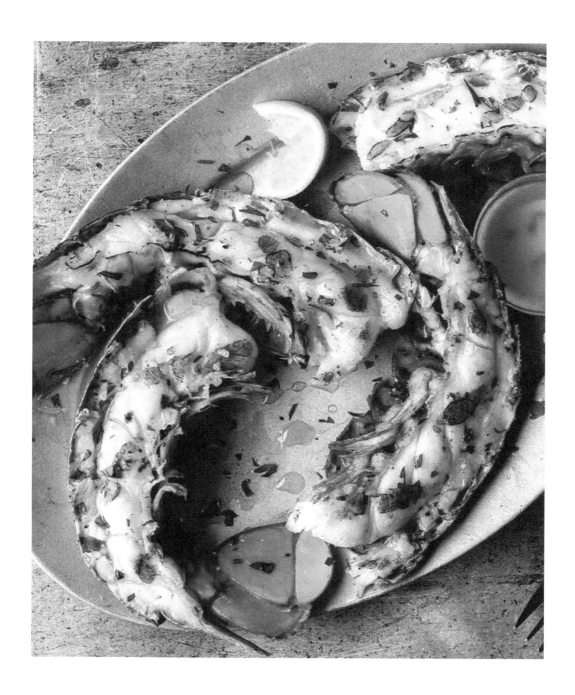

(Ready in about 15 minutes | Servings 4)

Per serving: 322 Calories; 26.5g Fat; 1.8g Carbs; 19.3g Protein; 0.7g Sugars

Ingredients

1 pound lobster tails 1 tablespoon Creole seasoning blend Lime Cream Sauce: 1 stick butter 2 tablespoons shallots, finely chopped 1/4 teaspoon salt 1/4 teaspoon black pepper 1/4 teaspoon cayenne pepper 2 tablespoons lime juice 1/4 cup heavy cream

Directions

Prepare the Instant Pot by adding 1 ½ cups of water and a steamer basket to the bottom of the inner pot. Place lobster tails in the steamer basket. Sprinkle with Creole seasoning blend. Secure the lid. Choose "Manual" mode and Low pressure; cook for 3 minutes. Once cooking is complete, use a quick pressure release; carefully remove the lid. Wipe down the Instant Pot with a damp cloth. Now, press the "Sauté" button and melt the butter. Now, add the shallots, salt, black pepper, and cayenne pepper; cook for 1 minute and add lime juice and heavy cream. Cook until the sauce has reduced. Spoon the sauce over the fish and serve right now. Bon appétit!

Beer-Poached Alaskan Cod

(Ready in about 10 minutes | Servings 4)

Per serving: 310 Calories; 23.5g Fat; 2.7g Carbs; 17.9g Protein; 0g Sugars

Ingredients

1 pound Alaskan cod fillets 1/2 cup butter 1 cup white ale beer 1 tablespoon fresh basil, chopped 1 teaspoon fresh tarragon, chopped 2 garlic cloves, minced 1 teaspoon whole black peppercorns 1/2 teaspoon coarse sea salt

Directions

Add all of the above ingredients to your Instant Pot. Secure the lid. Choose "Manual" mode and Low pressure; cook for 3 minutes. Once cooking is complete, use a quick pressure release; carefully remove the lid. Serve right away. Bon appétit!

Haddock and Cheese Stuffed Peppers

(Ready in about 15 minutes | Servings 3)

Per serving: 352 Calories; 20.1g Fat; 7.6g Carbs; 35.3g Protein; 3.6g Sugars

Ingredients

3 bell peppers, stems and seeds removed, halved 3/4 pound haddock fillets. Flaked 1 cup Romano cheese, grated 4 tablespoons scallion, chopped 2 garlic cloves, minced 4 tablespoons fresh coriander, chopped 1 tablespoon ketchup Sea salt and ground black pepper, to taste 1 teaspoon cayenne pepper 1/2 cup tomato sauce 1 cup water 2 ounces Pepper-Jack cheese, shredded

Directions

In a mixing bowl, thoroughly combine the fish, Romano cheese, scallions, garlic, coriander, ketchup, salt, black pepper, and cayenne pepper; mix to combine well. Now, divide this mixture among pepper halves. Add 1 cup of water and a metal rack to your Instant Pot. Arrange the peppers on the rack. Top each pepper with tomato sauce. Secure the lid. Choose "Manual" mode and High pressure; cook for 10 minutes. Once cooking is complete, use a natural pressure release; carefully remove the lid. Lastly, top with Pepper-Jack cheese, cover and allow the cheese to melt. Serve warm and enjoy!

Authentic Garam Masala Fish

(Ready in about 15 minutes | Servings 4)

Per serving: 159 Calories; 7.4g Fat; 4.7g Carbs; 18.1g Protein; 2.2g Sugars

Ingredients

2 tablespoons sesame oil 1/2 teaspoon cumin seeds 1/2 cup leeks, chopped 1 teaspoon ginger-garlic paste 1 pound cod fillets, boneless and sliced 2 ripe tomatoes, chopped 1/2 teaspoon turmeric powder 1/2 teaspoon garam masala 1 ½ tablespoons fresh lemon juice 1 tablespoon fresh parsley leaves, chopped 1 tablespoon fresh dill leaves, chopped 1 tablespoon fresh curry leaves, chopped Coarse sea salt, to taste 1/4 teaspoon ground black pepper, or more to taste 1/2 teaspoon smoked cayenne pepper

Directions

Press the "Sauté" button to heat up the Instant Pot. Now, heat the sesame oil. Once hot, sauté the cumin seeds for 30 seconds. Add the leeks and cook an additional 2 minutes or until translucent. After that, add the ginger-garlic paste and cook for 40 seconds more. Add the other ingredients and stir to combine. Secure the lid. Choose "Manual" mode and Low pressure; cook for 6 minutes. Once cooking is complete, use a quick pressure release; carefully remove the lid. Bon appétit!

Red Curry Perch Fillets

(Ready in about 10 minutes | Servings 4)

Per serving: 135 Calories; 4.1g Fat; 1.3g Carbs; 22.3g Protein; 0.6g Sugars

Ingredients

1 cup water 1 large-sized lemon, sliced 2 sprigs rosemary 1 pound perch fillets Sea salt and ground black pepper, to taste 1 teaspoon cayenne pepper 1 tablespoon red curry paste 1 tablespoons butter

Directions

Pour 1 cup of water into the Instant Pot; add the lemon slices and rosemary; place a metal trivet inside. Now, sprinkle the perch fillets with salt, black pepper, and cayenne pepper. Spread red curry paste and butter over the fillets. Lower the fish onto the trivet. Secure the lid. Choose "Manual" mode and Low pressure; cook for 6 minutes. Once cooking is complete, use a quick pressure release; carefully remove the lid. Serve with your favorite keto sides. Bon appétit!

Bluefish in Tarragon-Vermouth Sauce

(Ready in about 10 minutes | Servings 4)

Per serving: 204 Calories; 7.9g Fat; 4.4g Carbs; 23.5g Protein; 2.3g Sugars

Ingredients

2 teaspoons butter 1/2 yellow onion, chopped 1 garlic clove, minced 1 pound bluefish fillets Sea salt and ground black pepper, to taste 1/4 cup vermouth 1 tablespoon rice vinegar 2 teaspoons tamari 1 teaspoon fresh tarragon leaves, chopped

Directions

Press the "Sauté" button to heat up the Instant Pot. Now, melt the butter. Once hot, sauté the onion until softened. Add garlic and sauté for a further minute or until aromatic. Stir in the remaining ingredients. Secure the lid. Choose "Manual" mode and Low pressure; cook for 3 minutes. Once cooking is complete, use a quick pressure release; carefully remove the lid. Bon appétit!

King Crab with Baby Bellas

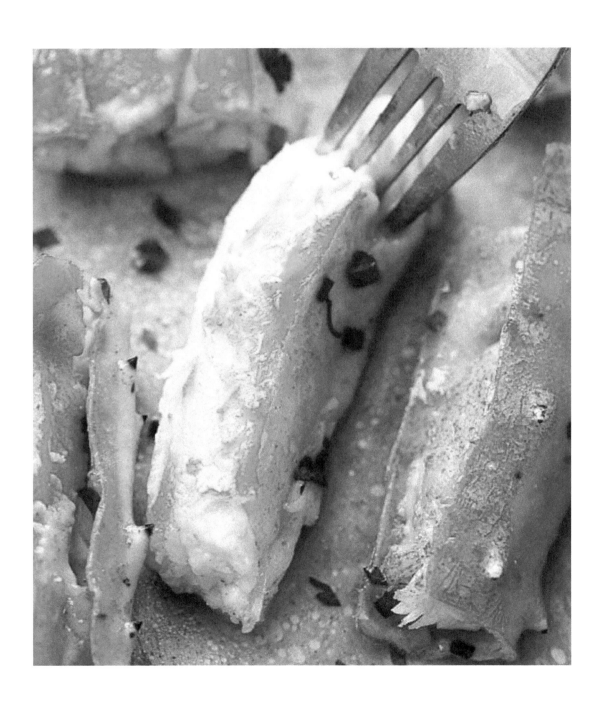

(Ready in about 10 minutes | Servings 6)

Per serving: 176 Calories; 8.5g Fat; 2.4g Carbs; 22.3g Protein; 1.1g Sugars

Ingredients

1 ½ pounds king crab legs, halved 1/2 stick butter, softened 10 ounces baby Bella mushrooms 2 garlic cloves, minced 1 lemon, sliced

Directions

Start by adding 1 cup water and a steamer basket to your Instant Pot. Now, add the king crab legs to the steamer basket. Secure the lid. Choose "Manual" mode and Low pressure; cook for 3 minutes. Once cooking is complete, use a quick pressure release; carefully remove the lid. Wipe down the Instant Pot with a damp cloth; then, warm the butter. Once hot, cook baby Bella mushrooms with minced garlic for 2 to 3 minutes. Spoon the mushrooms sauce over

prepared king crab legs and serve with lemon. Bon appétit!

Simply Creole Sea Scallops

(Ready in about 10 minutes | Servings 4)

Per serving: 163 Calories; 4.7g Fat; 6.1g Carbs; 22.6g Protein; 0g Sugars

Ingredients

2 teaspoon butter, melted 1 ½ pounds sea scallops 2 garlic cloves, finely chopped 1 (1-inch) piece fresh ginger root, grated 1/3 cup dry white wine 2/3 cup fish stock Coarse sea salt and ground black pepper, to taste 1 teaspoon Creole seasoning blend 2 tablespoons fresh parsley, chopped

Directions

Press the "Sauté" button to heat up the Instant Pot. Now, melt the butter. Once hot, cook the sea scallops until nice and browned on all sides. Now, stir in the garlic and ginger; continue sautéing for 1 minute more or until fragrant. Dump the remaining ingredients, except for the fresh parsley, into your Instant Pot. Secure the lid.

Choose "Manual" mode and High pressure; cook for 1 minutes.

Once cooking is complete, use a quick pressure release; carefully

remove the lid. Serve garnished with fresh parsley and enjoy!

Salmon Steaks with Garlic Yogurt

(Ready in about 10 minutes | Servings 4)

Per serving: 364 Calories; 21.2g Fat; 4.2g Carbs; 37.2g Protein; 3.3g Sugars

Ingredients

2 tablespoons olive oil 4 salmon steaks Coarse sea salt and ground black pepper, to taste Garlic Yogurt: 1 (8-ounce) container full-fat Greek yogurt 2 tablespoons mayonnaise 1/3 teaspoon Dijon mustard 2 cloves garlic, minced

Directions

Start by adding 1 cup of water and a steamer rack to the Instant Pot. Now, massage olive oil into the fish; generously season with salt and black pepper on all sides. Place the fish on the steamer rack. Secure the lid. Choose "Manual" mode and High pressure; cook for 4 minutes. Once cooking is complete, use a quick pressure release; carefully remove the lid. Then, make the garlic yogurt by whisking Greek yogurt, mayonnaise, Dijon mustard, and garlic. Serve salmon steaks with the garlic yogurt on the side. Bon appétit!

Hangover Seafood Bowl

(Ready in about 15 minutes | Servings 6)

Per serving: 280 Calories; 14g Fat; 9g Carbs; 32g Protein; 2.8g Sugars

Ingredients

1 ½ pounds shrimp, peeled and deveined 1/2 pound calamari, cleaned 1/2 pound lobster 2 bay leaves 2 rosemary sprigs 2 thyme sprigs 4 garlic cloves, halved 1/2 cup fresh lemon juice Sea salt and ground black pepper, to taste 3 ripe tomatoes, puréed 1/2 cup olives, pitted and halved 2 tablespoons fresh coriander, chopped 2 tablespoons fresh parsley, chopped 3 tablespoons extra-virgin olive oil 3 chili peppers, deveined and minced 1/2 cup red onion, chopped 1 avocado, pitted and sliced

Directions

Add shrimp, calamari, lobster, bay leaves, rosemary, thyme, and garlic to your Instant Pot. Pour in 1 cup of water. Secure the lid. Choose "Manual" mode and Low pressure; cook for 3 minutes. Once cooking is complete, use a quick pressure release; carefully remove the lid. Drain the seafood and transfer to a serving bowl. In a mixing bowl, thoroughly combine lemon juice, salt, black pepper, tomatoes, olives, coriander, parsley, olive oil, chili peppers, and red onion. Transfer this mixture to the serving bowl with the seafood. Stir to combine well; serve well-chilled, garnished with avocado. Bon appétit!

Mussels with Tomatoes and White Wine

Ingredients for 2 servings:

1 tbsp extra-virgin olive oil 1 tbsp unsalted butter or extra-virgin olive oil 1 shallot minced 3 garlic cloves minced ¾ cup grape or cherry tomatoes quartered ½ tsp dried thyme ¼ tsp fine sea salt ½ cup dry white wine 1 cup seafood or fish stock 2 lbs mussels in the shell scrubbed clean 1 tbsp chopped fresh flat-leaf parsley Whole-wheat sourdough bread toasted, for serving

Directions and total time – 15-30 m

• Select the Sauté setting and heat the oil, butter, shallot, and garlic for about 4 minutes, until the butter is melted, the shallots are softened, and the garlic is bubbling but not browned. Add the cherry tomatoes, thyme, and salt and sauté for about 2 more minutes, until the tomatoes are slightly softened. Add the wine, bring to a simmer, and cook for about 3 minutes, until most of the wine has evaporated. Pour in the stock and bring to a simmer.

Add the mussels to the pot, discarding any that do not close to the touch, and stir to coat them in the cooking liquid. • Secure the lid and set the pressure release to Sealing. Press the Cancel button to reset the cooking program, then select the Pressure Cook or Manual setting and set the cooking time for 2 minutes at low pressure. (The pot will take about 10 minutes to come up to pressure before the cooking program begins.) • When the cooking program ends, perform a quick release by moving the Pressure Release to Venting. Open the pot. Spoon the mussels into a large, shallow serving bowl, discarding any that failed to open. Pour the cooking liquid over the top. • Sprinkle with the parsley and serve right away, with the bread on the side for soaking up the cooking liquid.

Scampi Shrimp

Ingredients for 4 servings:

¾ cup dry white wine or dry vermouth 2 tbsp butter 2 tbsp olive oil 4 tsp peeled and minced garlic ½ tsp dried oregano ½ tsp red pepper flakes 2 lbs frozen peeled and deveined raw medium shrimp 30-35 per pound

Directions and total time – 15-30 m

• Mix the wine, butter, oil, garlic, oregano, and red pepper flakes in an Instant Pot. Stir in the shrimp and lock the lid onto the pot. • Option 1 Max Pressure Cooker Press Pressure cook on Max pressure for 0 minutes with the Keep Warm setting off. • Optional 2 All Pressure Cookers Press Pressure Cook or Manual on High pressure for 0 minutes with the Keep Warm setting off. The vent must be closed. • Use the quick-release method to bring the pot's pressure back to normal. Unlatch the lid and open the cooker. Pour the hot shrimp and sauce into a bowl to serve.

Creamy Shrimp

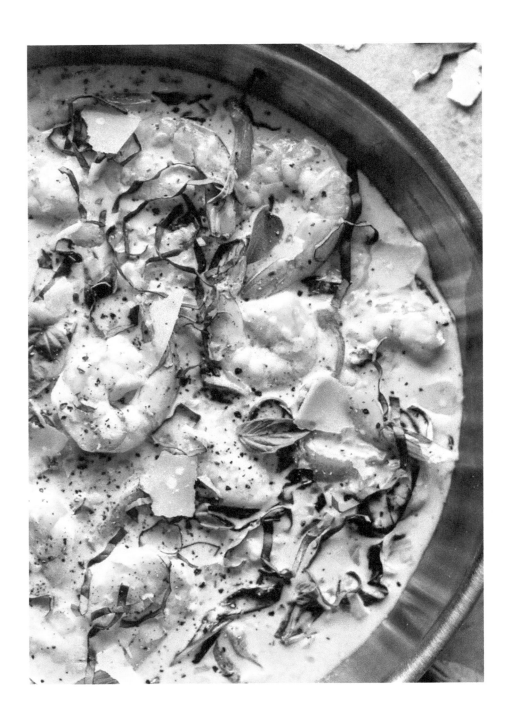

Ingredients for 4 servings:

1 lb peeled and deveined shrimp roughly chopped ½ tsp kosher salt ¼ tsp pepper 1 tbsp butter 1 tbsp olive oil ½ cup diced onion ½ cup diced celery 1 cup diced carrots 3 cloves garlic minced 2 tbsp brandy 1 ½ cups broth warmed 2 lbs tomatoes quartered ½ cup heavy cream 1 tbsp fresh chives snipped

Directions and total time – 15-30 m

• Season the shrimp with salt and pepper, then add butter to the Instant Pot. Using the display panel select the SAUTE function. • When butter melts, add shrimp and cook, tossing occasionally, until opaque throughout, 3 - 4 minutes. Transfer shrimp to a shallow dish and cover loosely with foil. • Add olive oil to the pot. When oil is hot, add onion, celery, and carrots to the pot and saute until softened, 3 - 4 minutes. Add garlic and cook for 1 - 2 minutes more. • Add brandy to the pot and cook for 30 seconds, then add broth to the pot and deglaze by using a wooden spoon to scrape the brown bits from the bottom of the pot. • Add tomatoes to the pot and stir to combine. • Turn the pot off by selecting CANCEL, then secure the lid, making sure the vent is closed. • Using the display panel select the MANUAL or PRESSURE COOK function. Use the +/- keys and program the Instant Pot for 8 minutes. • When the time is up, quick-release the pressure, then use an immersion blender to puree the soup. • Stir in heavy cream, adjust seasonings, then ladle the soup into bowls and top with the shrimp and chives.

Paella Pronto with Shrimp and Scallop

Ingredients for 4 servings:

Spice Mixture: 1 tsp paprika 1 tsp turmeric ½ tsp salt ¼ tsp black pepper ¼ tsp crushed red pepper 1 pinch saffron threads Shrimp and Scallop Paella Pronto: 4 tbsp butter 1 onion chopped 4 cloves garlic chopped 1 cup valencia rice or arborio 1 red bell pepper cut into short strips 1 cup chicken broth ½ cup white wine 1 lb large shrimp peeled and deveined (preferably 31-40 size or larger) 1 lb sea scallops 1 cup green peas frozen ⅓ cup chopped cilantro or italian parsley optional

Directions and total time – 15-30 m

Add butter to the Instant Pot. Using the display panel select the SAUTE function. 2. When butter has melted, add onion to the pot and saute until soft, 3-4 minutes. Add garlic and cook for 1-2 minutes more. 3. Add Spice Mixture ingredients to the pot and cook for 1 minute or until spices are fragrant. 4. Add rice and red pepper to the pot and stir well. 5. Add broth and wine to the pot and deglaze by using a wooden spoon to scrape the brown bits from the bottom of the pot. 6. Turn the pot off by selecting CANCEL, then secure the lid, making sure the vent is closed. 7. Using the display panel select the MANUAL or PRESSURE COOK function. Use the +/- keys and program the Instant Pot for 6 minutes. 8. When the time is up, quick-release the remaining pressure. Add the shrimp, scallops and frozen peas. 9. Cook and gently stir until shrimp and scallops are cooked through and most of the liquid has been absorbed, returning to SAUTE mode as needed. 10. (Optional) Arrange on a paella pan (or other wide, shallow, stovetop-safe pan) and set on the stovetop, uncovered, on medium-high heat until the bottom of the rice forms a crust, about 5 minutes. 11. Serve family-style sprinkled with cilantro or parsley.

Fish Tacos

Ingredients for 4 servings:

Amazing Fish Tacos: ¾ cup Water 4 6 oz tilapia halibut, or black bass fillets 1 tsp ground coriander 1 tsp dried parsley ½ tsp kosher salt ¼ tsp smoked paprika ¼ tsp pepper Topping Mixture: 4 Radishes thinly sliced ½ small cucumber halved and thinly sliced 2 tbsp fresh lime juice 2 tsp olive oil ¼ tsp kosher salt ¼ tsp pepper To Finish: 8 Corn tortillas warmed 1 cup fresh cilantro leaves ¼ cup sour cream Lime wedges

Directions and total time – 15 m

• Pour ¾ cup water in the pot. Place the fish in a steamer basket and season with coriander, parsley, salt, smoked paprika and pepper. • Lower the steamer basket into the pot, then secure the lid, making sure the vent is closed. • Using the display panel select the MANUAL or PRESSURE COOK function. Use the +/- keys and program the Instant Pot for 2 minutes. • Meanwhile, in a medium bowl, combine the Topping Mixture ingredients and toss to coat. •

When the time is up, quick-release the pressure. Check the fish for

doneness. If fish is not quite done, simply close the pot for a few

minutes and allow residual heat to bring to desired doneness. •

Serve the fish in tortillas with the cucumber relish, cilantro, sour

cream and lime wedges.

Clam Soup

Ingredients for 5-6 servings:

2 cups full fat coconut milk 2 bay leaves 1 cup grass-fed bone broth 1 pound cauliflower chopped 1 cup celery finely chopped ½ teaspoon freshly ground black pepper ½ teaspoon kosher salt 4 ounce small onion thinly sliced, ¼ onion 7 ounce clams chopped, 2 cans drained 1 cup heavy whipping cream

Directions and total time – 15 m

• Add the coconut milk, bay leaves, bone broth, cauliflower, celery, black pepper, salt, and onion to the Instant Pot. Stir thoroughly. • Close the lid, set the pressure release to Sealing, and select Manual/Pressure Cook. Set the Instant Pot to 5 minutes on high pressure and let cook. • Once cooked, let the pressure naturally disperse from the Instant Pot for about 3 minutes, then carefully switch the pressure release to Venting. Open the Instant Pot, remove bay leaves with tongs, and then stir in the clams and whipping cream. • Turn on Sauté mode, and let cook for 2 to 3 minutes (or until desired consistency).

Tostadas with Fish and Pineapple

Ingredients for 4 servings:

1 tbsp vegetable oil (approx.) 8 Corn tortillas 6-inch salt 20 ounces pineapple chunks, with juice 1 can ½ tsp hot pepper flakes ¾ cup Water 1-½ lbs skinless tilapia fillets cut into large pieces 1 cup deli-packed coleslaw 1 avocado cut into chunks (optional)

Directions and total time – 30-60 m

• Set your Instant Pot to Sauté on Normal. When the display says Hot, add 1 tsp oil, turning pot to coat bottom, and heat until shimmering. Add 1 tortilla and cook, turning once, for 2 minutes or until lightly browned. Transfer to a plate lined with paper towel. Season with salt. Transfer drained tortilla to a foil sheet. Repeat with the remaining tortillas, adding more oil as necessary between tortillas and stacking drained tortillas on the foil. Wrap tortillas in foil to keep warm. Press Cancel. • Set aside 2 tbsp pineapple juice. Add pineapple and the remaining juice to the pot. Stir in hot pepper flakes and water. Add tilapia on top, overlapping as necessary; do not stir. ● Close and lock the lid and turn the steam release handle to Sealing. Set your Instant Pot to pressure cook on Low for 3 minutes. ● When the cooking time is done, press Cancel and turn the steam release handle to Venting. When the float valve drops down, remove the lid. The fish should be opaque and should flake easily when tested with a fork. (If more cooking time is needed, continue pressure cooking on Low for 1 minute.) ● Meanwhile, stir reserved pineapple juice into coleslaw. ● Layer 2 tortillas, mostly overlapping, on each serving plate. Using a slotted spoon, spoon fish and pineapple onto tortillas. Top with coleslaw. Serve garnished with avocado, if desired.

Scallops and Tomato-Herb Sauce

Ingredients for 4 servings:

2 tbsp vegetable oil 1 medium red onion peeled and diced 1 clove garlic minced 3 ½ cups fresh tomatoes peeled 6 ounces tomato paste 1 can ¼ cup dry red wine 2 tbsp chopped fresh Italian parsley 1 tbsp chopped fresh oregano 1 tsp salt ¼ tsp black pepper 1 ½ lbs fresh scallops cleaned and drained Hot cooked pasta or rice (optional)

Directions and total time – 15-30 m

• Press Sauté; heat oil in Instant Pot. Add onion and garlic; cook and stir 3 to 4 minutes or until onion is soft and translucent. Add tomatoes, tomato paste, wine, parsley, oregano, salt and pepper; mix well. • Secure lid and move pressure release valve to Sealing position. Press Manual or Pressure Cook; cook at high pressure 8 minutes. • When cooking is complete, press Cancel and use quick release. Taste sauce; season with additional salt and pepper if necessary. ● Press Sauté; add scallops to pot. Cook 1 minute or until sauce begins to simmer. Press Cancel; cover pot with lid and let stand 8 minutes or until scallops are opaque. Serve over pasta, if desired.

Fish Stew

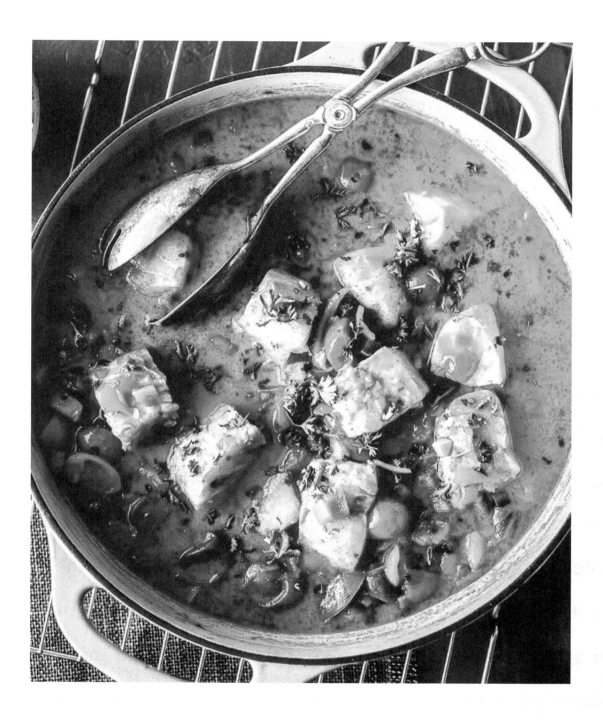

Ingredients for 1 serving:

2 tsp olive oil 1 clove garlic minced ½ cup onion chopped ½ red bell pepper cut into 2-inch pieces ½ green bell pepper cut into 2-inch pieces ½ potato a ½ tsp smoked paprika 1 cup chicken broth 4 ounce cod fillet 1 cod fillet (thawed, if frozen) 14.5 ounce diced tomatoes 1 can ¼ cup small cooked shrimp (thawed) 1 lemon wedge 1 tbsp fresh dill chopped ¼ cup fresh parsley chopped

Directions and total time – 15-30 m

• Turn the Instant Pot on. Choose the Sauté program and the Normal setting. Once it has come up to temperature, add the oil. • Add the garlic and onions and cook, stirring frequently for 3 minutes, or until they begin to soften. Add the peppers, potato, smoked paprika, chicken broth, and tomatoes. • Closed the lid and vent, set to Stew" and the temperature to Normal. Set the timer to 5 minutes. • Once the time is up, quick release the pressure according to the manufacturer's directions to release the steam. •

Open the lid and add the cod fillet, close the lid and the vent, set to Stew and the temperature to Less. Set the timer for 8 minutes. • When the time is up, quick release the pressure according to the manufacturer's directions. Open the lid and stir in the shrimp. Close the lid for 5 minutes to allow the shrimp to heat through. • Ladle the stew into a large bowl, garnish with herbs and lemon wedge.

Mussels Frites

Ingredients for 4-6 servings:

Frites: 1 tablespoon rosemary chopped fresh 1 ½ teaspoons garlic powder 1 teaspoon salt ¾ teaspoon black pepper 1 ½ pounds russet potatoes or gold potatoes, cut into ½ inch-thick sticks 3 tablespoons olive oil Mussels: 1 cup white wine 3 roma tomatoes seeded and chopped 2 cloves garlic minced 1 bay leaf 2 pounds mussels scrubbed and debearded ½ cup flat-leaf parsley chopped fresh Dipping Sauce: ⅓ cup mayonnaise 2 tablespoons roasted red pepper minced 1 clove garlic minced

Directions and total time – 30-60 m

• Preheat oven to 450°F. In a small bowl combine rosemary, garlic powder, salt, and pepper. On a large baking sheet or roasting pan toss the potatoes with the olive oil and spice mixture. Roast for 25 to 30 minutes or until tender and browned, stirring once. • Combine the wine, tomatoes, garlic, and bay leaf in the Instant

Pot. Top with the mussels. Secure the lid on the pot. Close the pressure-release valve. ● Select manual and cook at high pressure for 3 minutes. When cooking is complete, use a quick release to depressurize. ● Meanwhile, for the dipping sauce, in a small bowl combine the mayonnaise, roasted red pepper, and garlic. ● Top mussels with parsley. Serve the frites with the dipping sauce alongside the mussels.

Fish and Greens with Miso Butter

Ingredients for 2-4 servings:

1 cup vegetable or chicken broth 1 inch piece of fresh ginger peeled and cut into matchsticks 1 clove garlic sliced 2 white fish fillets such as tilapia (about 12 ounces total) 1 tsp soy sauce Salt and pepper 1 tbsp butter at room temperature 1 ½ tsp miso paste ¼ lemon 1 bunch kale tough stems removed and leaves torn (about 4 packed cups)

Directions and total time – 15-30 m

• ADD the broth, ginger, and garlic to your Instant Pot. Place the trivet on top followed by a piece of aluminum foil. Place the fish fillets, side by side, on top of the foil, drizzle with soy sauce, and season with salt and pepper. Secure the lid. • COOK at low pressure for 7 to 10 minutes depending on the thickness of the fillets and use a quick release. • MEANWHILE, make the miso butter: Mix the butter and miso well in a small bowl and set aside. • ONCE the pressure has released, check the fish for doneness and carefully remove using the foil. Squeeze lemon juice over the fillets. • CAREFULLY remove the trivet. Turn on the Sauté function and, once simmering, add the kale. Cook for 1 to 2 minutes, until wilted, and turn off the Sauté function. Remove using tongs or a slotted spoon. Season with salt and pepper. • TOP the greens with the fish fillets and serve with miso butter.

Cod with Panko-Crusted

Ingredients for 4 servings:

½ cup panko bread crumbs 2 tbsp extra-virgin olive oil 2 tsp grated lemon zest ¼ tsp salt ¼ cup light mayonnaise 2 tsp lemon juice ½ tsp dried thyme 4 cod fillets 6 oz, each about 3 inch or 4 inch thick 1 cup Water 1 lemon cut into 4 wedges

Directions and total time – 15-30 m

• Press the Sauté button, then press the Adjust button to "More" or "High." When the display says "Hot," add the bread crumbs and cook for 2 minutes, or until golden brown, stirring frequently. Stir in the oil, lemon zest, and salt. Remove from the pot and set aside on a plate. • In a small bowl, combine the mayonnaise, lemon juice, and thyme. Spread equal amounts over the top of each cod fillet. • Place the water and a steamer basket in the Instant Pot. Add the fish to the steamer basket, mayonnaise side up. Seal the lid, close the valve, press the Cancel button, and set to

Manual/Pressure Cook for 3 minutes. • Use a quick pressure release. When the valve drops, carefully remove the lid. Remove the steamer basket and fish from the pot. Serve the fish topped with the bread crumb mixture. Serve with the lemon wedges to squeeze over all.

Low Country Shrimp

Ingredients for 6 servings:

12 ounce beer or substitute same amount of water ½ cup Water 1 tbsp garlic minced 3 ears corn shucked and cut into thirds 1 ½ lbs red potatoes egg-sized 12-16 ounces kielbasa smoked sausage 1 package, cut into 2-inch pieces 1 tbsp cajun or creole seasoning (optional) 2 tbsp Old Bay seasoning, divided 1 ¼ lbs Shrimp medium to large 1 tbsp lemon juice ⅓ cup butter melted ½ tsp garlic powder Additional Old Bay for garnish (optional) Cajun seasoning for garnish (optional)

Directions and total time – 30-60 m

• Combine beer, water, and garlic in the pot. Stir to combine. • Add corn, potatoes and sausage. Sprinkle the cajun seasoning (if using) and 1 tbsp of the Old Bay and over the top. • Secure the lid, making sure the vent is closed. • Using the display panel select the MANUAL or PRESSURE COOK function. Use the +/- buttons and program the Instant Pot for 4 minutes. • When the time is up, quick-release the remaining pressure. • Add shrimp and sprinkle lemon juice and remaining 1 tbsp Old Bay over the top. Replace the lid and make sure the pot is still set to WARM. The residual heat will cook the shrimp. Check for doneness after 5 minutes. • Use a slotted spoon to remove corn, potatoes, sausage and shrimp to a serving platter. • Mix together butter and garlic powder. Pour butter mixture over the platter or serve on the side for dipping. • Garnish with additional Old Bay and/or cajun seasoning. Serve warm.

Soy-Ginger Dressing Salmon and Broccoli

Ingredients for 4 servings:

1 lb wild-caught Alaskan salmon. Cut into four 4-ounce fillets. Fine sea salt and freshly ground black pepper. SOY-GINGER DRESSING: 6 tbsp extra-virgin olive oil 2 tbsp soy sauce or tamari 2 tbsp raw apple cider vinegar 1 tbsp minced fresh ginger (about 1-inch knob) 1 clove garlic 3 tbsp pure maple syrup 1 tsp toasted sesame oil 1 lb Broccoli cut into florets sesame seeds for garnish Chopped green onions, tender white and green parts only for garnish

Directions and total time – 15-30 m

• Pour 1 cup water into the Instant Pot and arrange the handled trivet on the bottom. Place the salmon fillets on the trivet in a single layer, skin side down. Sprinkle them generously with salt and pepper. • Secure the lid and move the steam release valve to Sealing. Select Manual/Pressure Cook to cook on high pressure for 0 minutes. When the cooking cycle is complete, immediately move the steam release valve to Venting to quickly release the steam pressure. • While the fish is cooking, make the dressing. Combine the olive oil, soy sauce, vinegar, ginger, garlic, maple syrup, and sesame oil in a blender and blend until smooth, about 1 minute. Set aside until ready to serve. • When the floating valve drops, remove the lid and place the broccoli directly on top of the cooked fish. Secure the lid again and move the steam release valve to Sealing. Select Manual/ Pressure Cook to cook on high pressure for 0 minutes. When the cooking cycle is complete, immediately move the steam release valve to Venting to quickly release the steam pressure. • When the floating valve drops, remove the lid. Use tongs to transfer the steamed broccoli and salmon to serving plates. Drizzle the dressing over the top and garnish with the sesame seeds and green onions. Store leftovers in an airtight container in the fridge for 4 days.

Tomato Cod Fillets with Zucchini

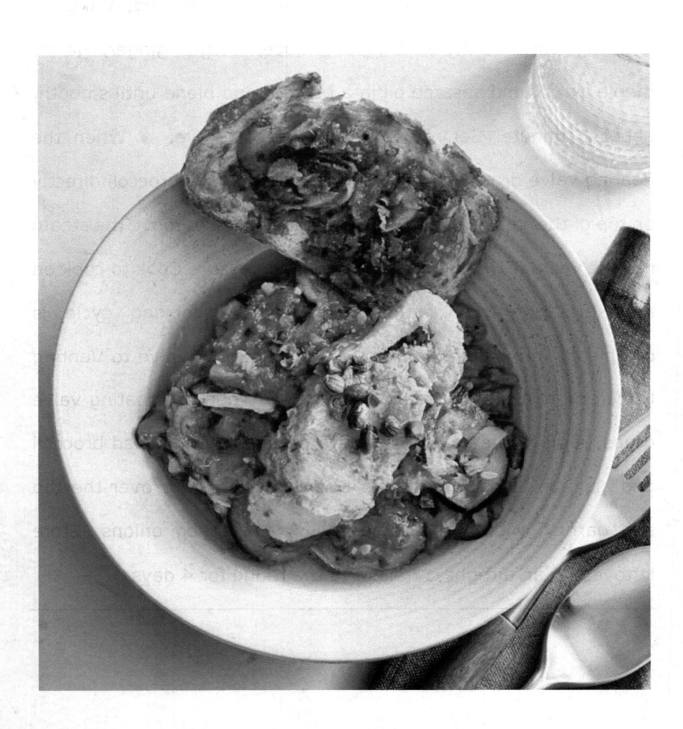

Ingredients for 4 servings:

28 ounces diced tomatoes packed in juice 3 ½ cups 10 ounces frozen sliced zucchini; or 1 medium zucchini sliced into ¼-inch-thick rounds, 2 cups ½ cup frozen chopped onion or 1 small yellow or white onion, peeled and chopped 4 ounce diced pimientos (1 jar); do not drain 1 tbsp dried Provençal or Mediterranean seasoning blend 4 frozen skinless cod fillets 6 ounces each

Directions and total time – 15-30 m

• Stir the tomatoes, zucchini, onion, pimientos, and seasoning blend in an Instant Pot. Lock the lid onto the cooker. • Option 1 Max Pressure Cooker Press Pressure cook on Max pressure for 3 minutes with the Keep Warm setting off. • Option 2 All Pressure Cookers Press Pressure Cook or Manual on High pressure for 4 minutes with the Keep Warm setting off. The valve must be closed. • Use the quick-release method to bring the pot's pressure back to normal. Unlatch the lid and open the cooker. Nestle the cod fillets into the sauce. Lock the lid back onto the pot. • Option

1 Max Pressure Cooker Press Pressure cook on Max pressure for 5 minutes with the Keep Warm setting off. • Option 2 All Pressure Cookers Press Pressure Cook or Manual on High pressure for 6 minutes with the Keep Warm setting off. The valve must be closed. • Again, use the quick-release method to bring the pot's pressure back to normal. Unlatch the lid and open the cooker. Use a large cooking spoon to transfer the fish and sauce to serving bowls.

_____

Zucchini and Vegetable Tian

Ingredients for 4 servings:

1 tbsp olive oil ½ medium yellow onion peeled and diced 2 garlic cloves minced 1 cup Water 1 medium yellow squash cut into ½ inch-thick slices 1 medium zucchini cut into ½ inch-thick slices 2 roma tomatoes cut into ½ inch-thick slices 1 large russet potato cut into ½ inch-thick slices ¼ tsp salt ⅛ tsp black pepper ½ cup shredded mozzarella cheese ¼ cup grated parmesan cheese

Directions and total time – 30-60 m

• Press Sauté button on Instant Pot. • Add oil and onion. Let cook 4 minutes or until onion is soft. • Add garlic and cook an additional 30 seconds until fragrant. • Remove garlic and onion and spread in the bottom of a (7") cake pan. • Clean inner pot and place back inside Instant Pot. Add water and trivet to pot. • Arrange sliced vegetables in a pattern of squash, zucchini, tomato, potato around the edge of the cake pan. Continue in the center of the pan until the vegetables are all used. • Top with a paper towel and cover top of pan tightly with foil. Create a foil sling and carefully lower cake pan into Instant Pot. • Close lid and set pressure release to Sealing. • Press Manual or Pressure Cook button and adjust time to 30 minutes. • When the timer beeps, allow pressure to release naturally for 10 minutes. Quick release remaining pressure and then unlock lid and remove it. • Remove pan from Instant Pot using foil sling. Sprinkle salt, pepper, mozzarella, and Parmesan cheese on top. Serve warm.

Tabbouleh Vegetable Quinoa

Ingredients for 6 servings:

2 cups quinoa rinsed 3 ½ cups Water 1 tbsp extra-virgin olive oil 1 lemon juiced 1 English cucumber peeled and diced 2 medium tomatoes diced 4 scallions white and light green parts only, chopped ¼ cup chopped fresh flat-leaf parsley 2 tbsp chopped fresh mint ⅓ cup pine nuts toasted

Directions and total time – 30-60 m

• Combine the quinoa, water, olive oil, and lemon juice in the inner pot. • Lock the lid into place. Select Pressure Cook or Manual; set the pressure to High and the time to 20 minutes. Make sure the steam release knob is in the sealed position. After cooking, quick release the pressure. • Unlock and remove the lid. Using a fork, fluff the quinoa, then stir in the cucumber, tomatoes, scallions, parsley, mint, and pine nuts. • Serve immediately, or place the tabbouleh in an airtight container and refrigerate for up to 4 days.

Vegan Chili with 3 Beans

Ingredients for 6 servings:

Dry ingredients: 2 tablespoons chili powder 1 tablespoon smoked paprika ½ tablespoon ground cumin 1 teaspoon dried garlic ½ teaspoon sea salt ⅓ cup dried onion 2 tablespoons dried celery 2 tablespoons dried carrots 2 tablespoons diced dried mushrooms such as porcini or shiitake 2 tablespoons sundried tomatoes ½ cup dried black beans ½ cup pinto beans ½ cup great northern or cannellini beans For cooking and serving: 6 cups vegetable broth or water

Directions and total time – 30-60 m

• Preparation: Layer the dry ingredients in the jar in the order listed. • To Cook: Place all of the jarred ingredients into the Instant Pot. Add 6 cups of vegetable broth or water. Stir to mix. Cover with the lid and ensure the vent is in the "Sealed" position. Pressure Coo or Manualk on High for 40 minutes. Allow the steam pressure to release naturally for 20 minutes, then release any remaining pressure manually.
